CALORIE WARS:
Fat, Fact and Fiction

CALORIE WARS:
Fat, Fact and Fiction

LARRY DEUTSCH, MD
JEFF SCHWEITZER, PHD

LOGIC HOUSE PRESS
Spicewood, TX

ISBN 978-0-9847166-0-9

CONTENTS

INTRODUCTION

As with many projects, "Calorie Wars: Fat, Fact and Fiction" started with something personal. Larry contacted Jeff after reading his book "Beyond Cosmic Dice: Moral Life In A Random World." We got together to discuss the philosophy detailed in the book and soon realized that along with a shared interest in ethics, we had both been noticing a disturbing health trend in popular culture with increasing frustration.

That we need help is easy to see every time we walk down the street. The experts confirm what the obscured view in front of us tells us. They estimate that 64% of adults in the United States are obese and that this percentage is growing. Even our children are being affected, as nearly every one in three American children under the age of 18 is overweight. Associated with this weight gain are increased risks in adulthood for joint problems, angina, high blood pressure, heart attacks, strokes, type 2 diabetes and, ultimately, premature death. Outside of the human costs, health experts estimate that treating adult obesity-related ailments will cost the American economy nearly $150 billion in 2009.

Everywhere we look we see someone championing a "superfood" or complicated formula for losing weight. We each have our anecdotes of frustration. Jeff hit a wall of bias after submitting a blog to the Huffington Post detailing the fallacy of all diets based on anything other than calorie reduction. The editors there believed that the sage advice of "eat well, eat less and exercise" constituted "medical advice" that could only come from an MD, which was simply an excuse not to publish an article that challenged virtually every other blog on the site.

For Larry the epiphany came when standing captive in the checkout aisle at the supermarket. In front of him, in bright colors and eye-catching fonts was a women's magazine that promised to help readers "lose weight like a teenager," "crack your body's weight loss code", "lose 11 lbs a week," and encouraged them to "fill up on fat-burning super foods." A well-known doctor wearing a white lab coat over his shirt and tie smiled at Larry from the cover. "Is he really signing off on this?" Larry wondered, getting angrier as he thumbed through the magazine. "He knows better." Larry thought of all his patients and many others who might see the magazine and come away with the idea that by following Dr. Q's special diet they would be delivered from their weight loss problems. This was nothing but a modern version of snake oil, and a disgrace.

Rather than tapering off, the $40 billion-a-year weight-loss industry, bolstered by pseudoscience and wishful thinking, continues to ramp up. Magazines, books and diet gurus touting special fat-burning and metabolism-increasing foods and eating schedules are the rule rather than the exception. As a biologist and as a physician, we could clearly see the impact of this barrage of myth-disguised-as-science on the nation's knowledge base and health.

Most of us no longer believe in the Tooth Fairy. Yet we believe in the equivalent, as adults, when we accept the idea that we can lose weight by taking a pill or eating some superfood or by following the latest nutrition fad. Because most of us lack an understanding of how physics and biology dictate what happens in our bodies, we are easy targets for an industry trying to convince us to buy weight-loss programs no less mythical than exchanging dollars for teeth at night. Our general lack of knowledge has also allowed us to accept as food all kinds of engineered junk destined to make us fat, including many "health foods."

As a scientist, Jeff is concerned that pseudo-science has taken over the collective conscience, confusing the differences between basic terms like "calorie," "metabolism" and "fat-burning" as they are now commonly but incorrectly used. If the fundamental concepts are not understood, we can be easily exploited by official-sounding diet advice that is nothing but pure nonsense.

Having worked for over 30 years as a family doctor and hypnotherapist with patients trying to lose weight, Larry knows there are no shortcuts to lasting weight loss. The solutions themselves are not complicated, but for most of us losing weight takes time; creating a lifestyle that will keep us thin requires dedication. Having seen the powerful mind-body connection in action with hundreds of patients, Larry believes hypnosis can help identify unknown weight-loss hang-ups and reinforce healthier habits. But hypnosis is no quick fix. True liberation comes only when we rid ourselves of our ties to superfoods, fast weight loss and fad diets, and instead embrace a sustainable way of eating and exercising based on real science.

We've seen the toll these trends in weight gain have taken firsthand and felt an obligation to use what we've learned to explain the truths of weight loss and guide you toward healthful eating and exercise so that you, too, will have a real chance to lose weight and improve your health.

Fact and Fiction: Don't Be Fooled by Fad Diets and False Promises

Let's start out by being blunt: we're fat and it is killing us. We need to talk honestly about how we can decrease our girths and improve our health. If we hide behind euphemisms and false promises we will never make any progress. That is why this book is all about tough love: telling you the hard truth about losing weight that you might not want to hear. But it is real, and what we offer really works.

As such, this book is short. Our goal is to tell you everything you need to know, and not one thing more. We could easily pad the text to make this a 300-page tome. Instead, we stick to the most essential basic facts. This slim volume contains everything you need to lose weight and keep it off, and nothing extraneous to that specific goal.

We include here, too, some important myth busting to attack the worst, and most popular, diet claims. One prominent diet guru, for example, tries to explain "why a calorie is not a calorie." Run for the hills! This nonsense masquerading as science exemplifies everything that is wrong with the diet industry today. There aren't different kinds of calories, just as there aren't different kinds of degrees Fahrenheit. Fad diets try to defy physics with pseudo-science, but you can't fool Mother Nature.

If you learn one thing from reading this book, let it be that any diet promising results too good to be true is nothing but an empty promise meant to con you. Admit it: you've tried a dozen diets, and have eventually abandoned each one, often packing on more pounds than ever after the latest diet is just a bitter memory. You start each diet with renewed enthusiasm and commitment, so why don't they work? Herbal Magic, Zone, Atkins, South Beach, 4-Hour Body, Body Fat Diet, the list is almost endless, and so are the gimmicks, broken promises and silly fads. The reason for "serial dieting" is that weight loss has no easy answer, but that is nevertheless exactly what you are promised, and so each ultimately leads to failure.

Do not succumb to the seduction of the easy. There are *simple* answers, but no easy ones. That is the hard truth: losing weight and staying thin is not easy. Anyone telling you otherwise is selling you Florida swampland. Run away as fast as you can and keep your hand on your wallet.

You might object that you know friends who really lost weight following one diet or another. Let's be crystal clear about this: any diet works by altering your behavior in order to reduce your caloric intake. If eliminating carbs from your diet induces you to eat fewer calories, you'll lose weight. But that has absolutely nothing to do with avoiding pasta and rice; what you've done is found a way to reduce the total calories you consume.

So what is wrong with that? Nothing in itself, but we have yet to find someone who can avoid carbs for the remainder of his or her life; and when carbs come back in, so do the pounds. Fads fade, but calories stick. The answer instead is to find a healthy, sustainable way to reduce caloric intake so that staying thin is a natural and normal part of your daily life.

Have you noticed that almost every major diet to reach fad status includes compulsory supplements and meals? Are these items essential to reaching a healthy weight and maintaining it? Of course not. The diet industry makes a fortune training you to eat tasteless, manufactured food because they think you are not smart enough to eat real food and too lazy to cook for yourself or bag your lunch. The truth is, real food tastes much better than whatever special formula some guru or food giant corporation prepackages for you as a "convenience" or "time saver."

Are we really too busy to feed ourselves properly? No, what we are is too busy doing nothing much productive: texting, logging on to Facebook, babbling on our phones and watching TV. That driver weaving in the next lane is probably not urgently texting the hospital to prepare the OR for the next organ transplant. We confuse the immediate for the important. We confuse motion for action. We really do have the time to stop by the store and pick up some fresh fruit. It's simply a matter of setting priorities. We have time to live well, no matter how busy we are, because in the end living well takes no more time than living otherwise.

You can be fat or you can be thin; the choice is yours. This book is designed to help you make well-informed choices. Instead of supporting an industry selling junk science and snake oil, declare your independence, take control of your life and lose the weight you want. We show you how with some very simple advice that requires nothing from you but a real desire and dedication to slim down. But you must be willing to let go of the destructive fantasy that you can lose weight without working hard at it with a deep commitment to the end result. That is tough love, and that is the truth.

Rather than presenting restrictive diets that simply cannot be followed long term, our suggestions are geared toward helping you find a new, sustainable way of eating and exercising. While we aren't deprivation advocates, losing weight *will* require you to set some new boundaries around what you eat and do not eat. We hope that as part of choosing well, you will come to like and include many new foods that can substitute those you may have to set aside.

Our first chapter, The Basics, deals with the calorie and the science of weight loss. It is our hope that with a good basic understanding of what goes on in your body when you eat, you will be better able to tailor your eating and food choices to your weight-loss goals.

The next chapter, Before You Jump In, previews what to expect when you follow our suggestions, including *realistic* weight-loss time frames. Being realistic is one of the most important elements in creating lasting weight loss.

Since losing weight and staying thin requires some deep self-examination, this chapter also gives you some hard questions to ask yourself about your weight and what you plan to do about losing excess fat.

In the last chapter, Deprogramming Yourself, we introduce our rules: eat less, choose well, be active and restructure your relationship with food. These tools will help you focus on what you'll need to do to lose weight for good.

CALORIE WARS:
Fat, Fact and Fiction

THE BASICS

The Lowly Calorie

Everybody talks about calories, but we can think of no subject more prone to disinformation and misunderstanding. No word in our vocabulary has been more corrupted by pseudo-science and misguided beliefs. We must clean up this mess before discussing anything else related to weight gain. Fortunately, that is easily done.

A calorie is a unit of energy defined as the amount of energy required to raise the temperature of one gram of water by one degree.

We have to say the following to protect ourselves from attack by science nerds. All others, feel free to skip to the next paragraph to continue our point. Yes, we mean degrees Celsius at one atmosphere, and the gram calorie (or small calorie) versus the original definition based on the kilogram. Note that when discussing food energy the common unit is actually the kilocalorie, but the prefix is almost always dropped, so people say calorie when meaning kilocalorie. Also, the amount of energy required to raise water temperature depends on the starting temperature, making the definition vulnerable to variability. For the sake of simplicity, we mean calorie, not kilocalorie, and we assume that calorie is equal to 4.2 Joules.

Nowhere in the definition of a calorie is there any mention of the *source* of fuel needed to raise the temperature of one gram of water one degree. To heat the water you can use a BIC lighter, burn coal or torch banana peels. The only important thing is the total energy necessary to raise the water temperature by the specified amount. Burning one calorie is burning one calorie no matter what is being consumed by the fire.

Therefore, we come to an important conclusion: one calorie of carbohydrate is exactly equal to one calorie from fiber, which is precisely equal to one calorie from saturated fat. One calorie of fruit equals one calorie from a fudge bar. As a unit of energy, a calorie remains constant, always, across all foods.

Of course, if you consume one pound of fudge you will consume more calories than if you eat one pound of broccoli because calories are more densely packed into the sweet. But if you take a small nibble of fudge equivalent to one calorie or a big bite of broccoli equal to one calorie, you will have consumed one calorie whether that came from the vegetable or confection.

We pound home this point because the calorie concept is so pervasively misunderstood that any intelligent discussion of weight gain or weight loss typically goes downhill from there. Understand this fundamental point: when discussing weight loss (ignoring for the moment nutritional health), and weight loss alone, **the *source* of calories you consume does not matter**. The only thing that matters is total calories you eat, regardless of where they come from, compared to total calories you burn.

Breakfast in Bed — Calories and Timing

The important corollary of this truth is that *when* you eat does not matter, either. If you consume 2,000 calories in a day, it matters not whether you eat them all in one meal or in five smaller meals, all at breakfast or all at dinner or five minutes before bedtime. All that matters is total calories in versus total calories out. So why is eating a good breakfast important? We know from experience that people who eat a light, healthy breakfast more easily lose weight and keep it off. That is because eating a healthy breakfast helps us reduce the total calories we consume during the remainder of the day. Eating breakfast is a good behavioral ploy to help you eat less (fewer total calories in), but nothing more than that.

And now it's time to obliterate the biggest diet myth of all: that eating immediately before bed will result in weight gain (compared to eating those same calories at breakfast or lunch or snack time).

No. It. Will. Not. But, you might plea, aren't you going to gain weight because you will not exercise to burn off those calories after eating? Doesn't going to sleep right after eating impact the calories in-calories out equation? No and no. We repeat: The only thing that counts over any 24-hour period is the balance between the total calories you ate versus the total calories you burned. It doesn't matter when you start the clock on the time period you use to measure the total calories in versus total calories out, as long as you measure in and out during the same interval.

To make that point clearer, let's say looking over the past week, I consumed about 14,000 calories by averaging about 2,000 calories per day. If, during that same seven-day period, I burned 14,000 calories, I would not gain weight. Even if I consume my full daily dose of 2,000 calories in one big meal right before bed every night, I will not gain weight if I burn all 2,000 calories every day through normal activity. And I could take in 3,000 calories one day and 1,000 calories the next; as long as I consume 14,000 calories in those seven days to match my intake I will see no weight gain. When you eat does not matter. The laws of thermodynamics do not know or care *when* you had dinner.

No matter when you top off your car, you can only go so far on a full tank of gas. You don't get more miles per gallon if you fill up 30 minutes after leaving your garage. The number of miles you travel when fully fueled will not vary by *when* you put gas in your tank. If you try to consume more energy than is contained in one tank of gasoline before refueling, you will run out of gas; if you travel a distance under conditions that require less energy than the total energy contained in one gas tank, you will have gas left over. That will be true no matter when you filled the tank. *When* does not matter. The laws of thermodynamics do not know or care when you filled your gas tank.

There are, of course, plenty of good reasons not to eat a big meal before bedtime. You might get up to use the bathroom more during the night and therefore sleep less, or have trouble going to sleep due to the stimulation of having had a meal. All valid reasons to avoid such late consumption; but these have nothing to do with weight loss.

Here is what thermodynamics knows absolutely. If your energy intake (food calories) equals the energy (calories) you burn up by living, breathing, working and sleeping, you will not gain any weight. If energy in exceeds energy out, you gain weight, with the excess energy stored as fat. If energy in is less than energy out, you lose weight by consuming previously stored fat. There is no other formula. Nothing else matters concerning weight loss but the balance between the total calories you take in and total calories you burn.

As an active man of 170 pounds, I will lose weight if all I eat is 1,200 calories per day of rich, dark chocolate fudge. I would not be healthy, because I would not be getting the necessary vitamins, minerals, fiber and other essential nutrients for a balanced diet, but I would lose weight. And I would lose weight at exactly the same rate if I ate only 1,200 calories per day of Red Delicious apples. Or 1,200 calories of protein; or 1,200 calories simple carbohydrates; or 1,200 calories complex carbohydrates; or 1,200 calories of anything edible. Because 1,200 calories is always 1,200 calories, no matter the source. *Energy in versus energy out*; nothing else matters in determining weight gain or loss. Nothing. That is an indisputable fact of biology and physics.

Metabolism

For us to make it through a day, we must chemically convert energy stored in food into useful energy we can tap for vital functions like mowing the lawn, mating and watching reality television. Living things have the ability to take matter and energy from their environment and change it from one form to another. That process of conversion is metabolism. Plants convert sunlight and carbon dioxide to cellulose and sugars. Herbivores convert plants and their sugars to meat and movement through the process of digestion. Carnivores do the same favor to herbivores.

Inside our cells, metabolism happens through aerobic respiration that involves combining glucose with oxygen, which yields energy plus carbon dioxide and water as waste. For those who enjoy symmetry, this is the exact reverse of the reaction that takes place with photosynthesis, a process in which plants use the energy of sunlight to combine carbon dioxide and water into sugar and oxygen.

We usually think of respiration as breathing in and out. But biologists also speak of a different type, cellular respiration. Cellular respiration is the process of converting food energy (calories) into a specific form of energy that your cells can use (called ATP, which like any good fire, needs oxygen to burn). Let's see how this works, starting by reaching out for that big bowl of peanuts sitting on the coffee table.

Grab some goobers, chew and swallow. We're on our way. What happens next is that digestion breaks down food (catabolism) into molecules such as glucose and simple carbohydrates. Cellular respiration gets its fuel from this digestive process, taking the products of digestion and converting them into ATP. Some of that ATP is then used to make new molecules (anabolism) that you need to live.

Here is an easy way to look at this: You eat in order to convert food fuel (calories) into ATP through catabolism and cellular respiration. You breathe to give your cells the oxygen they need to burn ATP, to make your skin and bone through anabolism, and to power all the other essential functions of life. So, through metabolism (the processes of cellular respiration, catabolism and anabolism), your body converts the calories (energy) in the food you eat into an energy source it can burn (ATP), to make the molecules you need to live, and to power the muscles you need to move and breath, which brings in the oxygen that allows you to burn ATP made from the food you gathered and ate … and so the cycle continues.

Gaining and Losing Weight

The precise biochemical pathways your body uses to break down food molecules and rebuild them into the molecules you need to live are outrageously complicated, intricately choreographed, awesomely fine-tuned feedback loops. Many of you will recall from early college days the dreadful task of memorizing the citric acid cycle (or Krebs cycle), integral to carbohydrate metabolism. Fats, proteins and carbohydrates all have unique catabolic pathways. But do not let scientists or nutritionists bamboozle you with these complexities; they are not relevant to weight loss, regardless of how impressive we might sound when talking about acetyl coenzyme A.

So why the biology lesson? Note that in describing how your body converts food calories to ATP, no mention was made of where those calories came from. Because ATP could care less if the calorie came from fudge or fruit. It takes so many units of energy (calories) to create an ATP molecule, whether those calories come from organic wheat or gooey processed sugar. So let us emphasize here again, when discussing weight loss alone, ignoring for the moment nutritional health, **the source of calories you consume does not matter.** We only care about calories in versus calories out.

Think of your body as a machine, albeit one that is extraordinarily complex. Like any machine we require energy to run. Let's say you require 2,500 calories per day to generate enough ATP to fuel your activities and to make all the supporting materials your body needs. Eat 2,500 calories per day and your weight will remain unchanged. Chow down on 4,000 calories per day, and 2,500 will be used to support all of your biological needs, and much of the remaining excess 1,500 calories will be converted to adipose tissue as storage for future use (aka fat). Munch only enough to bring in 1,000 calories a day, and your body will convert the energy stored in your fat reserves to manufacture enough ATP to fill the 1,500-calorie deficit. Bingo: You lose weight.

Factors That Affect Your Weight

Genetics

The inherited factors that affect our weight include our body composition and our satiety response. If our parents were muscular, we may be as well, and because muscle burns more calories than fat, we may be slim or slimmer than those people who inherited less muscle mass. In addition, some of us are genetically blessed to have a satiety meter that is extremely sensitive and stops us from feeling hunger when we have eaten enough, so that we do not over-consume. Another group is genetically predisposed to eating more before the satiety meter goes off. This group is also more genetically predisposed to being overweight.

*The most important thing to understand is that your genetic predisposition, whether fat or thin, is not a destiny. You can do something about it.

Calories

Caloric intake (food) is just part of the equation. Burning calories through activity, whether it is casual (fidgeting), involuntary (breathing) or through formal exercise, is the other part of the equation.

Hormones

There are a small number of people who have a hormonal condition (such as hypothyroidism) that makes losing weight more difficult. They are, however, not exempt from the calories in-energy out equation. If anything, their condition means that they need to focus even more intently on consuming fewer calories in order to beat obesity.

While it is statistically unlikely that you suffer from a hormonal condition that creates an obstacle to weight loss, tests for such conditions are now fairly easy to schedule. If you are concerned about having a hormonal condition, talk with your doctor to find out more.

Medication

Some medications can make you hungry by changing the satiety meter in your brain or in other biological pathways. Others can decrease your appetite. If you think a medication you are taking is affecting your eating habits, you should discuss this concern with your physician.

Smoking

As a physician, Larry is often asked whether quitting smoking will cause patients to put on pounds. Smoking is an appetite suppressant, so it may indeed be helping some smokers stay slim. However, smoking isn't a viable weight-loss tool, as it is one of the worst things you can do for your health. Cancer, heart disease, impotence and obstructive lung disease are just some of the negative effects of smoking that greatly overpower any appetite-curbing benefit it may give you. The good news is that you can learn to disconnect from smoking without substituting eating as your comfort behavior and gaining significant amounts of weight. In fact, Larry has helped many patients quit smoking through relaxation and hypnotherapy (see http://www.drlarry.com) without losing control of their weight.

How Many Calories Per Day

Figuring out the number of calories per day you need to lose weight will take some trial and error. The numbers we provide here are estimates as we cannot know your personal activity level. If you find that you are not losing weight with the number you select, go lower, being careful not to go below 1,200 per day without your physician's go-ahead and supervision. Keep in mind that you should never feel as if you are starving yourself. If, for instance, you find that you are losing weight at the number you selected but are constantly distracted by hunger, consider increasing the number of calories by 50-100.

Sedentary Women 1,500 calories per day

Sedentary Men 1,600 calories per day

Moderately Active Men and Women 1,700-1,800 calories per day

High Activity Men and Women 2,000 calories per day

Super High Activity Men 2,500-2,550 calories per day

BEFORE YOU JUMP IN

What to Expect

"Slow and steady wins the race." The hare in Aesop's classic tale discovered this truth when looking at the backside of a turtle. As you start to reduce your calories, increase your activity level and restructure your life to lose weight, you too may come to the same realization. Since we are advocating a sustainable new way of being rather than some drastic lettuce and water diet, your weight loss may be slower or less linear than you initially expect. The numbers on your scale may shift downward gradually or fluctuate from day to day instead of taking a consistent dive down. Don't let yourself get frustrated. This isn't uncommon as you embrace new habits and regimens.

Veterans of instant-gratification diets may want to know why our moderate approach may not result in immediate and dramatic (if temporary) results. In short, we aim for the long-term. Unlike the proponents of dramatic diets, we focus on losing body fat rather than muscle or water.

Here again a look at the science is helpful. Roughly speaking, there are three body constituents that are important when we speak about size and weight loss: water, body fat and muscle. Water, which comprises about 70% of your body weight, is found in every cell in your body. Body fat, made up of individual fat cells, can be found in larger deposits on the thighs, buttocks and abdomen; and less visibly as a kind of cushion around your organs.

Your muscles not only support your frame and facilitate movement, they also enable you to burn those all-important calories so critical to weight loss. When you go on a starvation diet, you often lose water weight and can, more disturbingly, lose muscle mass instead of body fat. This quick loss of water (and even muscle) can trick you into thinking that you are making a lasting difference to your size and weight. You may instead be setting yourself up for slower weight loss as well as a rebound in weight once you go off the diet.

Your body converts carbohydrates you eat to a substance your muscles can store for later use called glycogen. Carbohydrates must be paired with water to convert them to glycogen. When you first go on an extreme diet, your body releases glycogen to burn first-level reserves. Glycogen is reconverted to a carbohydrate (glucose) that your muscles can consume, and in the process water is released and the numbers on your scale go down.

While losing water weight may seem great, water loss can hide the fact that you may not be depleting body fat. But that is not the only problem. While a little counter-intuitive, water in fact is your friend when trying to shed pounds, not your enemy; water plays a crucial role in normal body function and weight loss. When you increase your activity level, your muscles store more glycogen (a process that requires water) in order to keep up with your new physical requirements. In addition, increased activity can result in increased blood volume (which requires water), in order to deliver more oxygen to your muscles, which in turn allows you to burn more calories.

Reducing body fat and building muscle should be your goals if you are trying to slim down. As muscle burns more calories than fat, the higher your muscle mass the more calories you use up, even at rest. When you think you are doing absolutely nothing, your body is actually engaged in a lot of hidden activities (including blinking, breathing, circulating blood, growing and repairing cells, adjusting hormonal levels, maintaining body temperature and all the other functions that keep you alive). Basal metabolic rate is the term used to describe the number of calories your body uses to perform these basic bodily functions. Sixty to 75% of the calories you use up each day are associated with your basal metabolic rate.

Factors that determine your basal metabolic rate:

Your body size and composition: Larger people and those with a larger amount of muscle mass burn more calories.

Your Sex: Men tend to have more muscle mass and less body fat than women of the same age and weight, so they burn comparatively more calories at rest.

Your Age: As we age, our body composition tends to change. The muscle component of our weight decreases and more of our weight can be attributed to fat, so our calorie burning at rest decreases.

Of course, you cannot change factors such as your height and gender, but you can work to increase your muscle mass and decrease your body fat, which leads to burning more calories.

The twin goals of reducing body fat and increasing muscle mass are accomplished by exercising and ramping down calories. Muscles, which are so important to burning calories, thrive when we use them.

Exercise, even of the casual kind, is what works your muscles. To really make strides with weight loss, you need to commit to increasing your activity level. Without a commitment to getting active, you are addressing only one part of the weight-loss equation.

Pacing Yourself

Rather than looking for immediate results, we want you to start to think long-term. Chart your progress at 14-day intervals for three-month periods. These time frames should allow you to lose weight at a sustainable pace. If your weight or shape does not change modestly after the first 14-day interval, it is likely you have not created the necessary calorie deficit through exercise and dietary change. To measure your progress, pick a pair of slacks, jeans or a belt that has been too tight for you to wear comfortably and notice that at every 14-day interval they fit better and better. Keep that success in mind every time you are tempted to fall back to the old habits.

Talking to Yourself

So far we've been dealing with weight loss on the physical level, describing the natural laws and processes that govern your size. Scientific understanding is important, but mental preparation and personal motivations are just as critical for long-term weight-loss success. Before you can begin your weight-loss journey, you will need to ask yourself some hard questions and make some firm resolutions.

The aim of the following four questions is to help you examine your inner life, your motives, and the memories and emotional responses that may be contributing to keeping you fat. You may want to work your way through these questions with a notebook in hand so that you can jot down your responses for later reference.

Why am I overweight?

This question is an invitation to examine as objectively as possible the factors that have led to and maintained your weight gain. Is it a matter of habits? What is your activity level? Does your extra weight have an emotional component? Is your weight connected to how you feel about yourself?

What behaviors and habits contribute most to me being overweight?

Little things add up. Maybe you habitually make your BLT with butter and mayonnaise. It could be that you have a large glass or two of wine with each lunch and dinner. Maybe you put cheese on everything and have dessert with every meal. Perhaps your pastimes are all sedentary; maybe you routinely and absentmindedly eat in front of the TV or computer. Do all of your social gatherings involve heavy eating and tippling? Do you work shifts and catch your (often fast food) meals as you can? Are convenience and restaurant meals your friends since you never learned to cook or feel you don't have the time to do so? Are the dishes you learned from your grandmother more suitable to your ancestors' lives of heavy labor than to your light activity level? Are stewing and frying meats common in your kitchen? Do you prefer to drive even when the distance is walkable? Do you automatically choose the elevator over the stairs?

If I've lost weight in the past, why haven't I been able to maintain that weight loss?

An event as simple as a holiday or a birthday celebration may have precipitated your return to obesity. Or maybe you regained the extra weight because you got a more sedentary job, your schedule changed or you suffered an injury or bout of depression. Perhaps you rebounded to being overweight because you found sticking to a diet too difficult and resigned yourself to being a larger size. Maybe you found yourself losing confidence in your ability to stay slim. Knowing what caused past failures will be important in order to move ahead and find lasting success.

Do I want to lose weight?

This isn't a trick question. We know you are reading this book because you have at least some interest in weight loss. But to actually lose weight you have to have more than just an interest in the topic. You must be totally committed. Expect success via hard work and commitment and let go of your fear of failure.

Some readers, even though they know that their energy levels and health would improve if they lost weight, are so fearful of failure they would have to answer "no" to this question.

Others would honestly have to answer "no" because they have become comfortable with the protection that their extra weight provides. They fear, at an unconscious level, how life would change if they became active, attractive, trim and sexy. Still others might give lip service to wanting to lose weight, but deep down are not willing to believe sustained weight loss is possible or that they deserve to shed the extra pounds.

Getting Past Obstacles to Losing Weight: Mary's Experience

Mary is a 42-year-old married suburban mom with two young children. She came to Larry as a patient after years of yo-yo dieting had left her frustrated. At 5'4" and 200 pounds, she was tired, discouraged and felt very unattractive. Although the meals she prepared for her family were healthful and the portions reasonable, she still wasn't able to slim down. On top of a fairly sedentary lifestyle, Mary had become a secret snacker. She was a frequent doughnut shop customer and avid baker. Sweets and late night cookies ostensibly baked for the family were comforts to her.

Larry began by encouraging Mary to do some psychological self-examination. In talking with him, Mary came to realize that she had never been able to imagine herself thin. Larry worked with Mary to create a mental image of herself as a lighter, healthier woman. She looked forward to more energy, the joy of movement, better sex, and a new wardrobe. She was determined to transform this image into reality.

With hypnosis, two changes were amplified. First, Mary would learn to cope with her stress without resorting to food as comfort and salvation. Second, using frequent and positive self-talk coupled with a new self-image, she could safely return to the trim, healthy woman she once had been.

Through hypnotherapy, Mary learned to still the voices that sabotaged her and to develop positive suggestions she could give herself when tempted to reach for a sweet or to cheat. Mary found hypnosis very relaxing, and it proved to be a powerful weight-loss aid for her. No longer was stress a trigger to overeat.

After six months of exercise and sensible eating supported by a hypnotherapy CD Larry created to target her issues, Mary was able to slim down to 140 pounds. Without an examination of what was really going on behind her obesity, Mary may not have been able to make the changes to her life that are necessary for lasting weight loss.

The hypnotherapy CD Larry created presented Mary with imagery, visualization, meditation and direct suggestion that helped her stick to our four simple weight loss rules and change old habits.

Since all suggestions require commitment and reinforcement, frequent relaxation with the CD was necessary to help Mary create new habits and attitudes. She learned to say "No thank you," to poor food choices and extra helpings and to postpone sweet cravings until the urge passed or lessened. She was also, more crucially, able to release her fear of change and improve her self-esteem and confidence.

DEPROGRAMMING YOURSELF

Since we've all been brainwashed by the diet industry for so long, we need to cleanse ourselves and clear our minds if we want to take a different approach to weight loss. Think of this as deprogramming similar to what cult members undergo to find their way back to society. The first step is to reject any and every diet that emphasizes or eliminates one food category like carbohydrates or proteins. Next reject any and every diet that requires you to take supplements, pills, oils, powders or body cleansers. These are all unnecessary and by not addressing your lifestyle and the behaviors that keep you fat, may actually be counter-productive. Finally, follow the four simple rules to eat less, eat well, be active, and develop a healthy relationship with food. Sounds simple. But the question is, how?

In the next section we provide you with practical steps you can take to lose weight and keep it off. If you are comfortable taking on the task of losing weight by yourself, using our four simple steps as your guide, we encourage you to get started now. If, after reading our step-by-step approach to weight loss, you think you might need help, consider Larry's self-hypnosis weight loss CDs. By no means is this approach the only one, or the only answer. Not everybody needs self-hypnosis to succeed, and not everybody will be successful doing it. But most will.

Weight loss is a matter of changing your behavior and daily routine so that in the end you consume fewer calories and modify your relationship to food. With self-hypnosis, you remain in control as you tackle this simple—but not easy—assignment. Larry is one of the pioneers in the field of weight loss and self-hypnosis and has been treating patients successfully for decades. If our advice resonates with you, but you are not sure how to get started, Larry's CDs and MP3s (see http://www.drlarry.com) offer guidance, structure and proven support.

Three Simple Rules, Plus One

In translating weight loss facts to a practical plan, we have found it useful to present our suggestions as rules. Use them as guidelines to losing weight.

- Rule One: Eat Less

- Rule Two: Choose Well

- Rule Three: Get Active

- The Final Rule: Restructure Your Relationship to Food

Rule One: Eat Less

As you start your weight-loss journey, eat smaller portions than you normally would. Whether you choose well or not (see Rule Two), eating less is a great way to create the calorie deficit necessary for weight loss.

"How much less?" you may ask. The word less refers specifically to calories. Assume you typically consume 1,800 to 2,000 calories to maintain your current weight. If you persuade yourself to consume 10% to 20% less food for most of your meals, without pigging out at the others, that creates a daily deficit of about 200 calories. If you are consistent and disciplined in your Eat Less commitment, then on average you would lose about two to three pounds weekly, even without significantly changing your activity level. The key here is consistency. Eat less nearly every day without letting up on whatever exercise you normally do, and you will lose weight.

Satiety — Stop Sign

We have many clues to when we should stop eating. Every one of us has a unique satiety system in our brain that tells us when we are full. We also have a hunger system that drives us to find food. These two systems have biological and genetic roots. Naturally skinny folk often have a sensitive satiety meter while those more prone to weight gain have a more sensitive hunger meter. Often the signal has little to do with actual hunger and more to do with social convention. Who does not want to try that free doughnut or those gooey sweets left in the office at holiday time? Who wants to refuse the pie that Auntie Peggy slaved over to make just for you?

We could write a large and quite boring book about the complexities of these multiple and competing hardwired biological and neuro-psychological systems. But such a tome is unnecessary because we need not let these complexities obscure a simple point: We can eat less in portion or calories if we want to.

Portion Alert

The food industry hasn't made it easy for us to choose reasonable portions. The portion sizes on offer continue to increase. Witness the bagel: time was that this common breakfast bread measured about three inches in diameter. Today's scaled up bagel comes in at about 6 inches in diameter. Three inches in diameter is now the standard cookie size, up from about one and a half inches in diameter. Muffins, another breakfast favorite, too have grown, from about the size of an egg to a monstrous standard of around 5 ounces.

All this super-sizing means that we need to focus on calories all the more. It won't cut it to continue eating four cookies if those cookies are now three times larger than they were in the past.

We need to be wary of the portion sizes of ready-made foods; when we encounter what we think are inflated portions we must be willing to reduce the amount we eat to suit the giant-sized dimensions. Here are some solutions for scaling down Goliath-size portions:

- Eat half or a quarter of that large bagel, sandwich, muffin or slice of pie, share the rest with a friend or save it for another day.

- Limit yourself (in the case of large cookies or biscuits) to just one, and take your time in eating it, so that you are able to extract the most pleasure from the experience.

- Hollow out baked goods like bagels and muffins, discard the innards and eat only the outer portion.

- Investigate other options, whose portion sizes will be easier to judge, like fresh fruit or yogurt snack packs.

- If you can't trust the portion sizes on offer, plan ahead and bring food you have prepared yourself.

Replace that little, inner voice from childhood that says "clean your plate or no dessert" with this new mantra: less is best, seconds are avoidable; with food so abundant I can wait until my next meal or snack.

Reinforcement

How are you going to accept this new mantra at the deepest level of mind and actually live it? All new habits require consistent reinforcement and repetition. Many who have failed at losing weight on their own have found success through hypnosis.

By entering a relaxed state, you can more easily absorb and internalize positive messages. Larry's patient Elvira told him, like others he's worked with, that when she forgets to listen to her hypnotherapy CD she falls off the wagon.

In time, frequent repetition of your own mantra will solidify the new diet and exercise changes you are now committed to.

Tips to Help You Stay on Plan

Here are some simple tips to help you stick to the Eat Less rule:

Plan your meals: When you don't plan your meals, it is easy to get ravenously hungry, over-eat or eat calorie-dense foods. Planning ahead ensures you design good-sized meals that are packed with fiber and proteins, which can sustain you for four to five hours until the next meal. Before each and every meal tell yourself, "This is what I have chosen to eat. Might as well extract every atom of pleasure and delight from each bite because when this is gone, I am done until the next meal."

Eat less, more often: If you find that you go so long between meals that your hunger cravings drive you to eat more calories than you should, eating smaller meals more often is a good behavioral ploy to help control caloric intake. You'll need to make sure, though, that you are eating small enough portions to sustain the energy deficit you need to become trimmer.

Un-Supersize: At home, think small when dishing out meals, and stop eating before you feel stuffed. Scaling down your plates, bowls, cups and glasses can also help you control portion sizes at meals, as our dinnerware has become super-sized along with our foods. Choose restaurants where dishes are a normal size or share your selections with someone.

Eat most of your meals at home: At home you can control your portion sizes and what goes into your meals. At a restaurant, most people have more difficulty avoiding high-calorie foods and giant-sized portions. See our Resources section for helpful websites and tools to help you cook good food at home and find healthy options when you are away.

Drink water: Between juices, sodas and alcohol, it has become all too easy to drink yourself fat. Straight from the tap, water is the perfect hydrator and zero-calorie beverage. It is best consumed as water, not soda with added sugar or diet soda with added chemicals or sweetened green tea or bottled vitamin water. Water can help you to feel full and nix the hungry feeling that might actually be thirst in disguise.

Practice mindful eating: To eat less, be present and mindful when you eat. No more all-you-can-eat buffets. Enjoy each morsel of food. Put your fork down between bites. Resist multitasking while you eat. If you wolf down your food while watching TV, walking, checking your cell phone, reading email, calling friends or other common ways we multitask, you are likely to frustrate or miss the "stop eating" cue.

Disciplined eating is a new habit for many of us. Like all new habits, it requires daily discipline and consistent practice. But once you get the hang of the new behavior, eating less becomes easier and easier.

Rule Two: Choose Well What You Eat

We feel your pain. Like you, we are surrounded by baseless and contradictory advice on what to eat. Our goal is to offer clarity, keeping our suggestions simple and easy to follow.

Low-energy-density foods

We live in a world of empty nutrition. That means chips, candy, processed foods, cookies, energy bars, flavored water, soda pop and a thousand other items masquerading as nourishment. Make a pact with yourself: eat foods that primarily come from a garden, an orchard, the ocean, or a farmer's field. Avoid food made in a plant; eat a plant instead. Choose real food you like and shun the rest.

Start a program of consuming more fruits and vegetables, right now, today. Colorful vegetables are generally healthier than their pale cousins like white potatoes or white rice. Why are vegetables so important? Nearly every vegetable is high in fiber, low in fat.

Also, consuming vegetables does not produce an elevated insulin response, which for some patients frustrates fat loss.

The energy balance equation of calories in and calories out that we have talked about and emphasized remains dominant for everyone regardless of our own unique metabolisms. Energy-sparse foods like vegetables contain less energy per gram than foods with high energy density like cookies or chocolate or ice cream. Whenever possible, choose foods with low energy density. If you must have a less healthy choice, like ice cream, then focus passionately on controlling portion size. One small scoop is sufficient; no more double or triple scoops with a waffle cone.

Eat fiber, which gets you full before you can get fat. White bread is a poor choice compared to whole grain bread, which usually has higher fiber content. Yes, you can get fat eating a bushel of apples, a high-fiber low-energy-density choice, but chocolate chip cookies will get you there faster.

Choose whole fruit over juice. Most fruits are low in calories per gram because they have high water and fiber content. By contrast, juice tends to concentrate the fruit's sugar, eliminate fiber, and encourage more rapid consumption, an unfortunate trifecta for weight loss. The time naturally required to enjoy a fresh whole orange, and all of that natural fiber, will trigger the satiety meter sooner than gulping an 8 ounce glass of juice.

Boost Your Fiber Intake

Keep a store of beans, lentils and peas in your pantry. Legumes are top of the list of vegetables when it comes to fiber, and these are a particularly good choice because they are also high in protein and versatile in the kitchen.

Choose bread and bread products made with flour from whole, intact grains. Substitute whole wheat bread for that baguette, oatmeal over Cheerios, and whole wheat pasta over plain durum pasta.

- Swap brown rice for white.

- Breakfast on bran and whole grain cereals (All-Bran, Bran Flakes, Weetabix, Oat Bran Squares).

- Add cereal bran to creamy foods like yoghurt and cottage cheese.

- Eat the skins of fruits like apples and pears.

- Snack on whole citrus fruits, like oranges, tangerines and grapefruit, instead of juice.

- Embrace fiber-rich "grains" like quinoa and amaranth as breakfast cereals or as substitutes for rice and pasta in side dishes and salads.

- Eat more fibrous greens like broccoli, cabbage, beet greens, collard greens and spinach. Steam them so they retain their body and flavor.

- Add orange vegetables like winter squash, carrots and sweet potatoes to your plate.

ELMO

Speaking of juice, let's do breakfast. Daily. Studies of patients who have lost weight and kept it off reveal that eating breakfast is a key variable in their success. Now as we've explained, *when* you eat has nothing to do with total calories in versus total out. We know from experience, however, that people who eat breakfast more easily reduce the total calories they consume during the rest of the day. Eating breakfast is a good behavioral ploy to help you eat less.

Generally, providing you are disciplined, follow the ELMO rule: Eat Less, More Often. We again emphasize here the word less. Portions must be small or you will not create the energy deficit necessary to become trimmer. Hunger cravings from long intervals without eating can lead you to consume bigger portions and higher total calories later on.

Snacking

If you find that snacking is putting you over your caloric limits, one strategy is to cut snacks out all together. Another way to go would be to make sure that your snacks are small and, as with your other meals, include plenty of fiber, protein and complex carbohydrates.

Snack Suggestions

- An apple or pear with a stick of low-fat string cheese

- A dozen raw almonds and an equivalent amount of dates or raisins

- One cup of air-popped popcorn (experiment with salt-free seasoning mixes for flavor)

- One cup of berries with 1 oz of hard cheese

- A banana with two tablespoons of unsweetened nut butter

- A bell pepper, cut into strips, with 1 oz of hummus

- ¼ cup of trail mix

- A fruit and low-fat yoghurt smoothie

- 1 ½ cups of light carrot soup topped with a few avocado slices

Eat Mediterranean

Conventional wisdom has long recognized the health benefits of the traditional foods of countries around the rim of the Mediterranean Sea. The typical diet in the region includes fruits, vegetables, whole grains, beans and various seeds, along with olive oil and moderate consumption of alcohol.

Foods From the Mediterranean Pantry

Fruits and vegetables

apples	apricots	cherries	dates
figs	grapes	lemons	oranges
pomegranates	prunes	quinces	raisins
artichokes	beets	bell peppers	carrots
celeriac	chili peppers	cucumbers	eggplants
fennel	garlic	leeks	mushrooms
okra	onions	salad greens	spinach
squash	tomatoes	zucchini	

Proteins

eggs	lamb	poultry	rabbit
ham	sausages		

beans (e.g. fava, chickpeas, lentils, lima, lupin and white)

fish and seafood (e.g. cod, anchovies, sardines, squid, fish roe)

Carbohydrates

barley	bread	bulgur	wheat
corn meal	couscous	pasta	potatoes
rice	semolina		

Dairy

cheese (fresh and aged — sourced from cows, goats, sheep, donkeys and buffalo)   milk   yoghurt

Oils, fats, nuts and seeds

almonds	butter and clarified butter		chestnuts
olive oil	olives	pine nuts	pistachios
walnuts	sesame paste (tahini)		

Aromatic herbs and spices

basil	coriander	cumin	dill
mint	mustard	parsley	saffron
sumac	thyme		

Condiments

honey	vinegar	wine

While not proven conclusively, this diet also appears to offer some protection against diabetes, cancer, heart disease and perhaps dementia. Articles in the American Journal of Clinical Nutrition and the New England Journal of Medicine and many other epidemiological studies clinically support these conclusions.

Fortunately, dishes from this region are rich in variety and flavor and as the ingredients are easy to find, this diet is not difficult to replicate at home. You simply need to create a diet that emphasizes: whole grain breads and other cereals, beans, nuts and seeds and olive oil as an important source of monounsaturated fat, dairy products, fish and poultry consumed in low to moderate amounts, red meat eaten only rarely, eggs consumed no more than four times weekly and wine enjoyed in low to moderate amounts of no more than two to five glasses weekly.

Our Resources section offers more on Mediterranean diets and cuisine.

A wonderful tangent benefit from a Mediterranean diet is that the food tastes great; you are not sacrificing when you adopt this lifestyle.

Choosing Well In Summary

Choose real food and shun the rest: Eat foods that primarily come from a garden, an orchard, the ocean or a farmer's field.

Aim for a balanced diet: Question any diet that emphasizes one food group over another. You need them all to maintain your body's balance.

Boost your intake of fiber-rich foods: Fiber can help you feel full and eat less. Fiber-rich foods like most vegetables and whole grains also don't produce the elevated insulin response that for some people frustrates fat loss.

Eat low-energy-density foods: Energy-sparse foods like vegetables contain less energy per gram than foods with high energy density like cookies or chocolate or ice cream. If you must have a less healthy choice, then focus passionately on controlling portion size.

Eat high-protein foods: Because foods high in protein help you feel satiated, they may help you eat less.

Eat foods that you enjoy: Eating well while losing weight doesn't mean depriving yourself of pleasure. You can eat what you love in moderation while exploring new foods to find healthful nutrition that will give you as much of a reward as high-energy-density foods.

Behind the Curtain: How Diet Plans Achieve Results

It should be clear by now that we are not fans of diets. We feel it is important, however, that you understand how diets work, so let's take a look behind the curtain.

All popular diet plans use the same formula: **decreasing calories and focusing on satiety to help achieve weight loss**. Here is a run-down of the mechanisms used by some of the more popular plans:

Atkins Diet — This diet restricts calories by eliminating carbohydrates. Satiation on this diet comes from high-fat, high-protein foods (e.g. meats, dairy, eggs).

Dean Ornish Diet — This vegetarian diet trims calories by cutting fats (a calorie dense food choice) down to only 10% of the total number of calories you consume and by avoiding simple carbohydrates such as sugar and honey. Satiation on this diet comes from fiber-rich foods and complex carbohydrates, eaten in adequate portions. The Ornish diet plan also emphasizes exercise, meditation and stress management — factors that can influence eating patterns and weight loss.

Jenny Craig — The Jenny Craig diet limits your calorie intake by controlling your meal portions and suggesting low calorie foods. At the same time, the plan encourages dieters to increase exercise levels.

The Zone Diet — The Zone Diet advocates getting 40% of your calories from carbohydrates, 30% from fat and 30% from protein in order to create satiety. The diet's caloric thresholds help ensure that you eat less (for example, meals should contain a maximum of 500 calories). Regular exercise is recommended.

GI Diet — This diet encourages you to eat fewer calories by selecting foods low on the Glycemic Index (a register that ranks foods based on how quickly they are broken down into sugar in the body and released into the blood stream). Foods low on this scale take longer to digest and tend to be complex carbohydrates and foods high in fat, fiber and protein. Exercise is recommended for GI dieters.

Nutrisystem — The Nutrisystem plan monitors calorie intake by controlling portion size. You are kept satiated on this diet by eating low Glycemic Index foods (see GI Diet above). The plan also encourages exercise.

South Beach — The South Beach diet is a high-protein diet that works by restricting carbohydrates in order to reduce your calorie intake. Exercise is not an integral part of this plan though South Beach dieters are told that physical activity will make the diet plan more effective.

Weight Watchers — Weight Watchers helps you cut back on calories through its POINTS system and by selecting low calorie density foods (through their Core Plan). This diet also encourages you to exercise and change the way you think about food. It can work well for those who benefit from a system that makes weight loss into a game.

Rule Three: Get Active

Study after study has proven the tremendous health value, including that of weight loss, of exercise. As with diet, when it comes to fitness, we are flooded with exercise programs that tout their successes and promise you great results. No amount of wishful thinking will overcome this fundamental reality: there are no magic bullets or wonder pills that will substitute for exercise.

Let's simplify. We are butterballs in part because we sit too much. We watch an average of 27 hours of TV per week, sit at a desk, and rarely move. Remember that weight loss depends on calories you take in versus calories you burn. If you are sitting around burning few calories, you are significantly reducing how much you can eat in order to maintain your weight. But instead of reducing the calories we eat to match our lack of activity, we do the opposite; the more we sit around the more we eat. And we get fat.

You do not need to be stuck in this cycle. Ideally you would commit to about 40 minutes of activity daily. Walk to work, take the stairs instead of the elevator, use that exercise equipment that is gathering dust, or just dance around the living room with your kids. Swim, hike, jog, do something. Do anything to get started. If 40 minutes is too much, then do 10 minutes or five. Anything is better than nothing, and then build from there.

Bad Exercise?

While all exercise is good exercise in theory, there are some activities that tend to take a great deal of time while offering a minimal reward in terms of slimming down or improving cardiovascular health.

Examples include:

- Baseball/Softball (A lot of time is spent on the bench waiting to play.)
- Bowling
- Curling
- Fishing
- Hunting
- Golf

That being said, these activities do burn some calories and are preferable to sitting on the couch.

By contrast, the following exercises are real calorie burners:

- Swimming
- Kick-boxing
- Biking/spinning
- Zumba (a Latin-inspired dance workout)
- Jumping rope
- Aerobic step classes
- Running

A word of caution when it comes to exercise: Do not be too ambitious too early; be realistic about what you will be willing to do on a daily basis. Sticking to your new routine is even more important than the rigor of your exercises.

Once you establish good habits you can more easily build on those habits to create an ever-more effective program of activities that is fully incorporated into your daily life. If initially all you can commit to daily is walking in a circle for one minute, then do that. Once that becomes a true habit, then make it two minutes until that becomes your daily habit. Then three minutes, until one day you decide going for a long walk is easier than doing circles in your living room.

Don't Have Much Time? Go For Efficient Exercise.

When it comes to burning fat, all forms of exercise are not created equal.

Interval Training

Interval training alternates short bursts of high intensity activity with longer periods of rest and slower activity. Also called high intensity cardio or high intensity intermittent training (HIIT), interval training may help you burn fat more quickly when compared to some other forms of exercise.

The idea is to stimulate the so-called "afterburn" effect in which your body, post-exercise, burns more calories at rest or sleeping than it would after a workout of unvarying pace. The "afterburn" effect is meant to represent energy your body expends to return itself to its pre-exercise state. While all of this remains unproven, evidence suggests that, depending on the intensity and duration of the exercise, it can take anywhere from minutes to days for your body to recover to its resting state.

Some of the potential benefits interval training offers:

- Helping you push beyond a plateau if you have been working out regularly but have stopped seeing results.

- Increasing your speed and endurance, regardless of your choice of exercise.

- Dramatically improving your cardiovascular fitness and decreasing your resting heart rate, so that your heart pumps more efficiently.

Interval training, however, isn't for everyone. If you have high blood pressure, joint problems, or if you have or are at risk for heart disease or stroke, you should discuss interval training with your physician before attempting it, as the intensity of the workouts may be too much for your body to take.

Super Slow

Super Slow is a resistance training exercise protocol that focuses on building muscle. Because muscle burns more calories than fat tissue, the more muscle you build, the more calories you will burn, even when resting.

With Super Slow you work with a trainer one or two times a week for 20-minute sessions. During your sessions you will lift and lower weights very slowly (each repetition takes at least 10-12 seconds of lifting and 5-6 seconds of lowering) to the point of total muscle exhaustion. All movements are carried out slowly, carefully and deliberately.

Super Slow is most useful for those new to weight training, as it will help them ramp up quickly. Other forms of weight training may be necessary to push intermediate or advanced weight trainers further. See our Resource section for more on this exercise protocol. As with interval training, Super Slow is not for everyone. Consult your physician before embarking on it, or any, exercise protocol.

Build up slowly so that your ambition does not exceed your commitment. The most common mistake we see is an ambitious plan that is soon abandoned because the patient could not realistically stick to the program on a daily basis. Select an activity that you really, truly will do every day, even if it's just for a few minutes. Then build on that. More than any other behavioral quality, consistency in meeting a commitment is the key to weight loss success.

Move about, walk every chance you get, do some exercises at your desk. Buy a pedometer and log at least 10,000 steps per day. Naturally skinny people burn calories via NEAT (non-exercise activity thermogenesis). Translation: they fidget more (burn more calories) than heavier people. Learn to fidget! Stop sitting like a bump on a log for hours in front of a computer or TV screen. You can burn an extra 75 calories a day by simply walking up and down stairs (at least 10 flights ideally, but start slowly) and parking your car at the far end of the lot at work, school or the store.

Simple Ways To Get More Active

- Walk whenever possible, instead of driving or taking transit.

- Choose the stairs instead of an elevator or escalator.

- Fidget your way through your day — whether you spend it walking around or are desk-bound.

- Take up more active pastimes. Limiting television and online time can help.

The key concept here is consistency. Consistent activity will keep you trim in the long haul, more efficiently and effectively than becoming a weekend gym warrior or cardio queen.

Be your own personal trainer. Ask yourself what you can do on a daily basis to boost your activity without breaking your back or wallet. Once you decide, whether you walk, jog, dance, swim, go to the gym, whatever, then like the Nike ad says, "Just Do It!" And do it daily. Your weight will fall, your heart health will improve, and you will enjoy life more fully.

There are just no magic bullets or wonder pills that will substitute for exercise.

Getting and Staying Motivated

A sedentary lifestyle, a less than stellar athletic ability, and a fear of being seen in exercise clothes are just a few of the many stumbling blocks Larry's patients have revealed to him as reasons that they resist the Be Active rule. It's possible that you are completely unaware that these types of hang-ups exist for you. Larry helps patients move beyond blocks like these through his hypnotherapy sessions, freeing them to enjoy the simple pleasure of movement.

Larry often tells patients that "the battle of the bulge is won on the playing field of your mind." Knowing that you should exercise is different from internalizing the desire to do so. Larry's hypnosis audio focuses on exercise as a way to experience the joy of physical activity; a way to treat your body to movement of all kinds and to better health.

Repeated listening in a hypnotic state to these positive statements about exercise helps quiet the hang-ups and fears that might be keeping you from exercising while reinforcing its pleasures and benefits.

Once you reframe how you feel about exercise and movement, you can easily change your sedentary lifestyle and follow a new mantra: "Be active, be joyful, have fun. Get off the sidelines, stop watching and enter the game of life with movement."

Larry's patient Betty always felt left out because her cerebral palsy had disqualified her from participating in many sports. In her mid-fifties, and forty pounds overweight, she had lost confidence in her ability to be active and saw herself as someone who would be relegated to a sedentary life. She needed to address both her mind and body issues so she could get moving and improve her health.

Rather than launch into a complicated or intensive fitness program, Betty focused on simply making sure to move for 10 minutes per hour every day as best she could. Since music energized Betty and helped her stay motivated this was integrated into her movement time. She even brought in a Jimmy Buffet CD and danced to "Margaritaville."

Larry's hypnotherapy sessions focused on encouraging Betty to envision herself exercising and seeing exercise as something fun that she could do every day. Although you won't see Betty on Dancing with the Stars, Larry was able to help her discover the joy of movement. She lost the extra weight, had fun doing it and still follows the Be Active rule to stay slim.

Get Active in Summary

Here is a summary of what we just learned:

Commit to exercise: If 40 minutes a day is too much, then do 10 minutes or five or one. A commitment to do one minute of exercise every day, if you *will actually do that one minute*, is better than a 30-minute pledge that you won't meet.

Incorporate exercise into your daily routine: Move about, walk every chance you get, do some exercises at your desk. The key concept here is consistency. Consistent activity will keep you trim in the long haul.

Be your own personal trainer: Ask yourself what you can do (and stick to doing) on a daily basis to boost your activity level without breaking your back or wallet. Whether that's yoga, walking, biking, jumping on a trampoline or swimming, commit to it and do it daily.

Once you establish good habits, you can more easily build on those habits to create an ever-more effective program of activities that are fully incorporated into your daily life.

The Final Rule: Restructure Your Relationship With Food

Now is the time to reference the answers to the questions we asked in the Talking To Yourself section. Your responses will help you get an idea of how you need to start to restructure your relationship with food.

Here are some of the responses Larry has heard from his patients.

"I'm motivated by memories of good times, which always involved food."

"I'm tired most of the time and I respond to the hit I get from eating the way I might to alcohol or cocaine."

"When I'm bored, I eat."

"My kids/spouse/friends don't eat well and I just go along with that."

"I think about food constantly — it's a struggle not to."

"I can't tell the difference between other needs like thirst, the company of others and hunger."

Perhaps similar thoughts have caused you to develop little unconscious eating habits that lead to obesity. Identifying these beliefs and heading them off or substituting a positive behavior as they arise is a critical step toward controlling poor eating habits. For example, if you tend to slather butter onto your morning toast you could work on creating an inner voice to remind you that a little goes a long way or you could substitute apple butter for dairy butter. If you can't resist buying doughnuts on the way to work, maybe you can take another route to work or develop an inner script that focuses your attention on something else along the way that you can enjoy. Maybe you have been overeating because you feel stressed out and for you food is a comfort. In this case, you could concentrate on helping yourself to relax, so that you don't feel the urge to overeat.

If you're struggling with motivation and commitment, your subconscious mind may, in fact, be sustaining your desire to keep eating. You will only be able to achieve sustainable weight loss when you have internalized positive messages and addressed the thoughts and beliefs that have previously blocked you from making the commitment to losing weight. Dealing with the reasons behind why we are overweight can be difficult to do unassisted. Self-monitoring, visualization, meditation and hypnosis are just a few strategies to help you stay on plan.

Self-monitoring: Keep track of the foods you eat each day. This food diary (on paper or online) will help you stay abreast of the calories you eat. Using a pedometer or a tech tool like the FitBit tracker (http://www.fitbit.com) will similarly help you to measure your levels of activity. See Resources for more helpful fitness tools.

Visualization: Imagine yourself eating the foods in your plan and walking away from a sweet you would otherwise be unable to resist.

Meditation: Regular meditation can help reduce your stress levels so you no longer feel the need to soothe yourself with food.

Hypnosis: As a family doctor, Larry uses hypnosis and self-hypnosis to help patients who want to lose weight but who cannot change their unhealthy eating patterns on their own.

The fact is that if you reorganize your life so that you are not consuming more calories than you burn, then you will lose weight. However, without addressing the psychological reasons that sabotage our attempts to reach and maintain a healthy weight, our weight loss aspirations are bound to fail long term. With hypnosis, patients can comfortably examine their lives and discover the factors that are blocking success. Once this is understood, they are quickly able to make the changes necessary for permanent weight loss.

To change a habit, frequent repetition of the new behavior is required. In Larry's experience, patients respond to suggestions more powerfully when delivered through hypnosis or self-hypnosis. Think of it simply as a way to amplify your response to counseling dedicated to our four simple weight-loss rules.

There are no clucking chickens or barking dogs in Larry's office. He uses hypnosis daily with weight loss patients with excellent results because the patients are in total control of all suggestions. Outside the office, Larry's weight-loss hypnosis CDs assists patients by reinforcing repetition and new habits to stay with the program.

MYTH BUSTING: WHY OUR RULES WORK — AND OTHERS DO NOT

So there you have our three rules, plus one. But why should you listen to us? After all, dozens of experts will tell you that we are wrong. Popular diets insist that you can fool your body with supplements of leptin or acetyl CoA or by consuming "fat eating" or "fat burning" foods. Here is the word from the National Institutes of Health: "No food can burn fat. Some foods with caffeine may speed up metabolism for a short time, but they do not cause weight loss." Yet we continue to see gurus and experts sell the lie of fat-burning foods — along with all the other nonsense that masquerades as professional advice.

While we cannot address every myth out there, let us look at some of the more widely accepted but false ideas that have permeated our society.

Hormones and Hormonal Supplements

Before dismissing the claims experts make about hormone supplements, we need to understand that our bodies are a finely tuned balance of feedback loops that regulate our essential needs and functions. The most obvious example of this type of dynamic equilibrium is thermoregulation, your body's ability to maintain a nearly constant internal temperature in the face of widely varying air temperatures. You also maintain innumerable other physiological parameters within tight specifications, including glucose levels, oxygen, carbon dioxide, salts, pH concentration and water content. The body accomplishes this task of maintaining stability in a changing environment through negative feedback mechanisms, responding in a way that counteracts any direction of change.

Blood sugar levels offer a good example: When sugar levels become elevated, the pancreas secretes insulin, which accelerates the storage of glucose in liver cells in the form of glycogen, removing glucose from the blood. When sugar levels fall, the pancreas secretes glucagons, which help break glycogen back into glucose, increasing blood glucose levels. Protein production is controlled in a similar way.

Any attempt to alter these intricate and complicated feedback loops with a supplement will be largely unsuccessful and may indeed have unintended consequences. Don't be distracted by pseudo-science and fancy jargon. Fiddling with the immutable laws of physics is a fool's game. You will likely do more harm than good when messing with a balance humans have acquired through four billion years of evolution.

Yet diet gurus keep trying to pimp the system. One doctor with a big TV audience talks a lot about leptin and ghrelin. Leptin is a hormone (protein), one of many dozens, involved in the complex feedback loop between brain and blood that balances hunger and satiety. Only in very rare cases is a deficit of leptin a weak link in someone's hormone balance. Also, like many hormones, leptin serves multiple roles (including moderating the inflammation response), so taking it in excess for diet purposes would almost certainly have unintended consequences. Ghrelin is a peptide (small protein, one generally released by the stomach) on the other side of that balanced equation that helps stimulate appetite. These two proteins are not "at war" with each other, but are part of a finely choreographed dance to balance your physiological needs. Artificially supplementing one or suppressing the other is just asking for trouble for very little gain because there is virtually no independent reproducible evidence that an imbalance of these hormones is the primary or even minor cause of obesity in our population.

Fat but Fit

Biology is a science of averages in which we can see significant individual variability. While smoking hugely increases one's risk for lung cancer, not all smokers get the disease. Such outliers prove rather than refute the rule by emphasizing the rarity of the unusual. Indeed a small percentage of obese people do not exhibit some of the problems associated with being overweight — and this has led to the dangerous idea that you can be fat but fit.

While we can point to a few obese individuals who do not appear to be at increased risk for heart disease, that should offer no consolation to you. Just because Betty Sue won the lottery does not mean you will. On average obesity leads to an increased risk for a variety of ailments, and you have a greater chance of suffering from such diseases if you are obese. Most Americans die sooner than necessary by stroke, heart attack or cancer, and obesity increases your risk for all of these.

We know absolutely that obesity creates an increased risk of diabetes. In 1990 about 11 million Americans had type 2 (adult onset) diabetes, a disease of insulin resistance (a condition that commonly coexists with obesity); just nine years later the number was 16 million, or about 6% of all Americans. Then from 1999 to 2003 we saw a 41% increase in diagnosed diabetes. Since then obesity has ballooned to an astounding 64% of all Americans and the number of diabetics continues to explode. The insulin resistance syndrome associated with obesity has other dire consequences, including hypertension and the increased risk of atherosclerotic cardiovascular disease.

Another problem with "fat but fit" is simple mechanics. The human body evolved from a period of deprivation where food was scarce and difficult to obtain. Our ancestors were almost certainly lean. In any case, we are not engineered to bear excess weight on our joints. Obesity leads to arthritis and can lead you down the path to knee replacement not only because of the mechanical stress it can cause but because fat produces chemicals that attack cartilage. Think of it this way: If you stuff 20 people into a VW Bug, the suspension will wear out faster and the engine will have to work harder, ultimately reducing its useful life.

If you still believe fat can be fit, consider the following realities:

About 300,000 deaths per year are attributed to obesity; individuals with a body mass index (BMI) over 30 have a 50% to 100% increased risk of premature death from all causes compared to lean people with lower BMIs.

High blood pressure is twice as common in obese adults compared to those with a healthy weight; obesity is associated with elevated blood fat (triglycerides) and decreased good cholesterol (HDL).

A weight gain of only 11 to 18 pounds increases the risk of developing type 2 diabetes; over 80% of people with type 2 diabetes are overweight or obese.

Obesity is associated with an increased risk of cancer of the uterus, colon, gall bladder, prostate, kidney, and postmenopausal breast cancer.

Sleep apnea is more common in obese people. And some recent studies have indicated that a lack of sleep might impact hormone levels to a degree that could, indeed, cause weight gain.

Obesity during pregnancy is associated with a greater risk of birth defects, including spina bifida.

Every increase in weight of two pounds increases the risk of arthritis by 9% to 13%.

One final consideration on the idea of being fat but fit. Obesity affects quality of life through limited mobility, decreased physical endurance, and social, academic and job discrimination. While we know we should not judge a book by its cover, we all do. Yes, you should be comfortable with and love yourself for who you are; and you need not look like a fashion model. But that truth is no excuse for carrying around excess weight.

The raw fact is that life is easier and, yes, more fun, when you are trim. Sex is better (how often do you hear, "I wish I were fatter again so I could enjoy sex more?"). This is not a male or female concern; obesity is equally detrimental to both genders. Do not buy into the idea that an aversion to obesity is a feminist issue; it is a health issue. Ricky Gervais lost considerable weight and has noted how happy he is being thinner; Drew Carey lost 80 pounds and he beams in the photos of the reduced him; John Goodman lost close to 200 pounds and anybody can witness how much happier he is at the lower weight.

The idea of "fat but fit" is simply an attempt to justify rather than address a problem.

Low Fat Versus Low Calorie

Clever advertising has created the idea that low fat means low calorie. It doesn't. The two are not equivalent by any means. Pretzels are almost fat-free but high in calories, with 10 pretzels having about 225 calories and less than two grams of fat. A standard serving of non-fat cottage cheese (obviously low fat) has 104 calories. A cup of 1% milk has three grams of fat and 120 calories. A low-fat chewy chocolate chip oatmeal-raisin cookie has 90 calories and two grams of fat. Protein bars usually have something like 100 calories and three grams of fat. "Low fat" does not give you license to pig out; you are still consuming calories, and the only thing that matters for weight loss is calories in versus calories out. Sure, reducing your fat intake is healthy and should be encouraged; but don't fool yourself into thinking that reducing fat alone will help you lose weight.

Cholesterol-Free Versus Non-Fat

Foods advertised as having no cholesterol often imply that the claim also means low in fat (or calories). Not true. To see why we need to set the record straight about fat facts.

Cholesterol — A waxy fat-like substance made by the liver and then circulated in the blood by two distinct carriers: LDL (low density lipoprotein) and HDL (high-density lipoprotein). LDL takes cholesterol from the liver to the rest of the body; HDL takes cholesterol from the body back to the liver. That is why we consider LDL to be the "bad" cholesterol and HDL to the "good" kind. The cholesterol we eat has little impact on our blood cholesterol levels (but other fats do; see next).

Saturated Fats — These tend to be solid at room temperature and are typically found in animal fats and tropical oils. Saturated fats contribute the most to elevated blood cholesterol levels, particularly LDL (the bad kind). For the science nerds out there, the word "saturated" refers to the fact that the carbon atoms in the fat are bound to the maximum possible number of hydrogen atoms (the carbon is saturated with hydrogen). These are found in desserts, snack foods, cream, lard, bacon, fatty cuts of meat, chicken skin and coconut palm oil. In spite of claims otherwise, no good evidence supports the idea that saturated fats reduce leptin levels (and therefore delay the feeling of being full).

Unsaturated Fats (mono and poly) — These are generally considered to be "good fats," but remember they still contain calories! Both mono- and poly-unsaturated fats are liquid at room temperature. Monounsaturated fats start to solidify at refrigerator temperatures while polyunsaturated fats remain liquid at cold temperatures. These fats actually help the body reduce blood cholesterol. Monounsaturated fats are found in olive oil, of course, but also in canola and peanut oil, as well as in avocados and avocado oil. Polyunsaturated fats, the healthiest of the bunch, are found in oils of sunflower, sesame seeds, soy beans, corn, nuts and seeds.

Trans-Fatty Acids — These are created during a process called "hydrogenation" that manufacturers use to make vegetable oil more solid at room temperature to produce margarine or shortening. Manufacturers and restaurants use trans-fats because they are cheap and stable over a long period of time, in many different conditions. Using trans-fats ensures a long shelf life for a box of supermarket cookies (long beyond the point at which the butter or vegetable oil in other cookies would have gone rancid) and lets your favorite fast food restaurant keep using a single batch of oil in its deep fryer multiple times.

While they have been a boon for the food processing and fast food industries, trans-fats are not as kind to our bodies. Trans-fats elevate blood cholesterol, especially LDL (although not to the same degree as saturated fats), and also lower HDL, a double whammy.

Trans-fats are found in baked goods, fast food restaurants, cookies, crackers, cakes, French fries, onion rings and doughnuts and other foods that are deep-fat fried in partially hydrogenated oils or use shortening, margarine or partially hydrogenated oil as an ingredient.

Omega-3 Fatty Acids — This type of fatty acid is highly polyunsaturated (meaning good for you) and is found primarily in cold-water fish like salmon, mackerel and herring, and now in some fortified eggs.

Triglycerides — A fancy name for our body fats that contain, in varying proportions, saturated, monounsaturated and polyunsaturated fats. Of the three, only the saturated fat component will raise blood cholesterol levels.

So what does this have to do with confusing cholesterol-free and non-fat? You can now see that the claim of "no cholesterol" is nothing but an ad gimmick. First, cholesterol is only found in products derived from animals; therefore *all plant-based products are naturally cholesterol-free*, including fruits, vegetables, whole grains and legumes. Second, and worse, the cholesterol found in foods is not even the main problem; foods rich in saturated fats and trans-fatty acids increase blood cholesterol more than cholesterol itself! Focus on the types and quantities of fat in the food rather than on cholesterol. And don't forget the calories no matter what the fat content may be.

You need not sacrifice to remain healthy. A quarter-cup of cashews has zero cholesterol and contains more than one-third of the required daily intake of monounsaturated fats (a good kind of fat). In spite of the unfortunate fad against carbs, we know that whole grain breads, cereals, rice, pasta and other grains, dry beans and peas are high in fiber and low in saturated fats and calories; in other words excellent choices for folks watching their weight and nutritional health.

Brown Fat

Much has been made in the media about brown fat (brown fat (brown adipose tissue), but as Shakespeare said, this is much ado about nothing. In infants brown fat, which helps generate heat, makes up about 25% of body mass as a means of keeping babies from becoming hypothermic. Some remains in adults but as a much smaller percentage of body mass. The misplaced excitement comes from the fact that brown fat burns calories from "normal" fat (white adipose tissue). Scientists can in certain circumstances induce in mice the growth of brown fat, which is related to muscle tissue. But do not hold out hope this will help you lose weight one day. Uncontrolled growth of brown fat leads to a hibernoma tumor; and even if we could induce growth safely the impact on weight loss would likely be minimal.

Belly Fat

The diet industry loves to talk about belly fat, largely because it sounds good. Central obesity does not have the same ring. The beer gut or pot belly, and growing rear end, is a consequence of an accumulation of visceral fat, as opposed to fat that accumulates under the skin or interspersed between skeletal muscle. The promise to "lose belly fat" using the "belly fat workout" or more egregious, the claim to teach you how to "burn belly fat" or the "dangers" of belly fat are all a bunch of hooey. You can't preferentially "burn" visceral fat in your tummy versus your bum or arm or surrounding your organs. We all want a flat stomach, so that is where the marketers focus their dollars.

The media makes way too much of the dangers of certain body shapes, for example correlating a pear shaped body with a greater risk for heart disease, hypertension and diabetes. The truth is that any form of obesity creates a risk for those diseases and belly fat does so only incrementally more. The greater problem is obesity, not the particular form of obesity. Men tend to suffer from central obesity more than pre-menopausal women, because women's hormones preferentially deposit fat in the butt, thighs, hips and breasts. Following menopause women become more vulnerable to belly fat. But where the fat goes is less important than the presence of the fat in the first place.

Much is made of the role cortisol plays in belly fat, but once again we find ourselves inappropriately focusing on one hormone among many dozens. Cortisol, a steroid produced by the adrenal gland, is commonly known as the "stress hormone." It is indeed true that one effect of cortisol is to act in the presence of stress to increase blood sugar through glucogenesis, and simultaneously aid in the metabolism of fat, protein and carbohydrates. This helps prepare the body for the "fight or flight" response. But cortisol has dozens of other physiological effects, and attempting to create a meaningful relationship between the steroid and fat, let alone specifically belly fat, is simply misleading. But don't be fooled: Stress does not make you fat. Forget cortisol, and remember that consuming calories in excess of what you use makes you gain weight, not some isolated hormone.

Anti-Inflammatory Foods

Doctors who dispense medicine on TV and online tell us that we can lose weight and promote better health by eating "anti-inflammatory" foods. This is yet another gimmick of little use to a person serious about healthy weight loss. Some studies have pointed to a link between inflammation and obesity but they are of little practical benefit when it comes to losing weight. All of the foods touted as being helpful in reducing inflammation are, ironically, the very foods you should be eating for a healthy diet focused on weight loss: fish, vegetables, fruit, nuts and seeds. Forget the complications of leptin, resistin, adiponectin and inflammation-induced leptin resistance. Don't waste time trying to figure out where you can get "anti-inflammatory" isoflavones, lignans, carnosol, reservartrol and quercetin. Instead, eat a balanced diet and limit your caloric intake. It's that simple.

Age and Weight

Maintaining a desirable weight becomes ever more difficult with age. The primary reason is that our metabolism slows down with advancing years. Why? We tend on average to exercise less, which leads to muscle loss — and muscle burns more energy than other tissue. This creates a cycle of less exercise, leading to more muscle loss, leading to even less exercise, then more muscle loss … and an ever-slowing basal metabolism. So our lean body mass decreases and we burn fewer calories per pound of body weight than we did as young adults. This by the way is not inevitable; muscles in the elderly respond to weight training to the same extent as in the young. A Tufts University study showed that an eight-week program of strength training in a cohort of women ages 87-96 resulted in a tripling of strength and an increase of 10% in muscle mass.

But the reality is most of us reduce our exercise regime as we age. Our metabolism inevitably slows, but our eating habits do not adjust accordingly. We continue to eat the same calories we did when younger, but burn less than before. The old "calories in to calories out" ratio soon tilts in favor of excess weight. A myth among baby boomers is that they can exercise their way out of this dilemma in order to defy age and gravity. Exercise certainly helps, and should be encouraged, but alone will not solve the problem. Consider that one full hour of high impact aerobics will burn only about 400 to 500 calories (depending on several factors, including your weight). To put that in perspective, a Toll House chocolate chip cookie contains 108 calories; you need to exercise strenuously for an hour to break even for every four cookies you eat. While exercise is extraordinarily important to maintain good health, the only realistic solution is to learn to eat less if you want to lose weight.

Myth Busters Grab Bag

We cannot possibly hit all the myths if we stick to our pledge to make this book short. So we will reach into the grab bag of myths and note that none are helpful to you. Temperature can affect metabolism and appetite; but not enough to be an effective weight loss tool. Sex is great, and can temporarily raise levels of oxytocin; but there's no help there with weight loss. High fructose corn syrup is making us fat for the simple reason it is a concentrated form of calories. The only thing behind the grapefruit diet is a reduction in the calories you consume; claims about grapefruit and reduced insulin resistance are unsubstantiated, as are the appetite-suppressing effects of smelling a grapefruit. Any weight loss solution needs to be holistic and science-based.

In seeking to understand our bodies, we try to take the easy path and focus on one hormone or one protein or one food. That is like trying to understand how a Boeing 747 flies by taking apart the call button that summons the flight attendant. We are too complex for such simplistic reductionism. There is no magic bullet. There is no simple pill or wonder food that will help. No matter how badly we want to make things easy, our bodies tell another story. Any promise of effortless or easy weight loss is a lie.

We do our entire population an enormous disservice any time we shy away from this simple advice: eat well, eat less and exercise. Anything else is a scam. We must take personal responsibility for our own bodies. Except in the most extreme and extraordinarily rare case, any human that eats less, eats well and exercises will lose weight. If circumstances prevent exercise, then eating even less is necessary. This is reality. This is life. No amount of wishing for a miracle will make one appear.

CONCLUSION

If you remember anything from us, remember this: if you want to lose weight, the only formula that works is the simplest one: eat less, eat well and exercise. Remember that weight loss depends only on reducing the total calories you take in compared to the total calories that you burn. Health depends on the quality of those calories.

Eat less: Snack less often, eat slowly, reduce portions or pick full portions of lower calorie foods.

Choose well: Eat more fresh fruits and vegetables and less processed food; eat fiber and whole grains; drink water.

Exercise: Even 10 minutes per day is better than nothing at all; incorporate some form of physical activity that you can live with and stick to into your daily routine.

Restructure your relationship with food: Identify and address the psychological blocks that sabotage your attempts to reach and maintain a healthy weight.

It takes just one glance at a newsstand or lineup of cars at a drive-thru window to see how insidious and institutionalized our society's unhealthy relationship with food has become. And there's much more at stake here than vanity. Obesity has led to an alarming increase in serious illnesses such as diabetes and heart disease. What's more troubling is the pervasive pseudo-science and false promises that have undermined so many individuals' attempts to lose weight, including the many patients who enter Larry's office on a daily basis.

But here's the good news: together, we can dispel the myths and enter a healthier, happier age of wellness. Our hope is that this book puts us on that path, and that you take away some clarity, guidance and inspiration from these pages to meet your own weight loss goals and improve your health for the long haul. Good luck!

RESOURCES

Food

My Recipes
http://www.myrecipes.com

An expansive recipe site, where a large number of the recipes include nutritional information. The site's search functionality allows you to search for recipes by nutritional content.

Eating Well Recipes
http://www.eatingwell.com/recipes_menus

A site linked to a magazine of the same name and focused on healthful eating. Recipes include nutritional information.

Eating Well - Healthy Mediterranean Recipes and Menus
http://www.eatingwell.com/recipes_menus/collections/healthy_mediterranean_recipes

Healthful Mediterranean recipes that include nutritional information along with information on the benefits of the Mediterranean diet and guides to Mediterranean cooking.

Clean Eating Magazine Recipes
http://www.cleaneatingmag.com/Recipes.aspx

A large collection of recipes that include nutritional information.

Exercise

Going Super Slow (article)
http://www.newsweek.com/2001/02/04/going-super-slow.html

Super Slow Resistance Training (article)
http://www.unm.edu/~lkravitz/Article%20folder/superslow.html

Super Slow Zone
http://superslowzone.com

A franchise provider of Super Slow resistance training with centers throughout the United States.

My Yoga Online
http://www.myyogaonline.com/home

Streaming yoga classes - take a yoga class from the comfort of your home.

Ultimate Pilates Workouts
http://www.ultimatepilatesworkouts.com/System-Requirements.
aspx

Take a Pilates class anywhere you are connected to the Internet.

Online Tools

DailyBurn
http://dailyburn.com

Sign up for the DailyBurn fitness community (basic service is free) to track your weight, what you are eating, your workouts and even your sleep. Related DailyBurn services include customized training plans, detailed progress reports, the DailyBurn, Meal Snap and FoodScanner iPhone apps, and motivational games.

Fitbit
http://www.fitbit.com

Fitbit is a fitness tracker that can help you keep track of your level of activity and number of calories burned, as well as sleep patterns (if you wear the tracker at night). You can also monitor the food that you eat through its online interface.

Fit Orbit
http://www.fitorbit.com

Fit Orbit connects you via the Internet with a personal trainer of your choice and provides you with a personalized fitness and meal plan.

Foodzy
http://foodzy.com

Foodzy helps you keep track of what you eat by turning it into a fun game. Foodzy creates a personalized, points-based diet plan for you, which you can use to "compete" against friends and family members. You can even win badges for healthful eating.

My Fitness Pal
http://www.myfitnesspal.com

This online community takes the food diary concept up a notch. Its huge, growing database of foods (catalogued with their caloric and nutritional values) makes logging your food intake and calories easier. Through its exercise database, My Fitness Pal also lets you keep track of calories burned and is available as an iPhone and Android app.

Mobile Apps

Cardio Trainer
http://www.worksmartlabs.com/cardiotrainer/about.php

Cardio Trainer uses GPS to track your workout activity with its pedometer function. This Android app includes integrated music, a fitness game you can play with friends, voice notifications of calories burned and distance traveled, and a social aspect where you can cardio-compete against yourself and others.

Livestrong Calorie Tracker
http://www.livestrong.com/thedailyplate/iphone-calorie-tracker

A popular calorie tracker for the iPhone and iPad.

Meal Snap
http://itunes.apple.com/us/app/meal-snap-calorie-counting/id425203142?mt=8

Meal Snap is an iPhone app that makes keeping track of the calories you consume easy. Simply take a photo of your meal, and Meal Snap will identify the food and give you a caloric estimate. This functionality makes keeping track of the foods you are eating and their calories convenient and easy.

RunKeeper
http://runkeeper.com

RunKeeper was one of the first fitness apps designed for the iPhone, and it's now also available for Android. The free app uses GPS tracking to measure exercise (not limited to running), monitor heart rate, and keep tabs on your progress. RunKeeper's premium version lets friends and family monitor your exercise history (a motivator for some people) and offers additional analytics.

ACKNOWLEDGEMENTS

We are honored to acknowledge Elise Aymer for her adroit editing, masterful organizational skills and keen ability to keep us, the two authors, on track and on message. *Calorie Wars* is a better book as a consequence of Elise's expertise and guidance, and for that we are eternally grateful.

AUTHORS

Larry Deutsch, MD

http://www.drlarry.com

Dr. Larry Deutsch, ("Dr. Larry") is a family physician and hypno-therapist with over 35 years of experience and offices in Ottawa and New York City. He specializes in helping patients achieve optimum health. A leader in the area of hypnosis in medicine, Dr. Larry is a frequent speaker on the role of hypnotherapy in health at medical seminars throughout the world.

Dr. Larry began using hypnotherapy to help his pregnant patients achieve calm, natural childbirth. Once he saw the powerful results that hypnosis provided to expectant mothers, Dr. Larry expanded his hypnotherapy to address other health concerns including:

- Weight Loss
- Smoking Cessation
- Panic Attacks
- Stress
- Insomnia
- Anxiety
- Boosting Confidence

Dr. Larry's hypnosis audios, available at http://www.drlarry.com, guide you to relax, release pain, make desired lifestyle changes, and renew and heal from within. His goal is to use hypnosis to activate your own self-healing and self-correcting potential. His comprehensive catalog of hypnosis MP3s and CDs is available worldwide.

Dr. Larry is a graduate of Cornell University and Dalhousie University's Medical School.

Jeff Schweitzer, Ph.D

http://www.jeffschweitzer.com

Dr. Jeff Schweitzer is a neurophysiologist, consultant and internationally recognized authority on ethics, conservation and development. He is the author of five books, including *Calorie Wars: Fat, Fact and Fiction*, and *A New Moral Code*. Dr. Schweitzer is a Huffington Post contributor and speaks regularly at science conferences worldwide.

He served at the White House during the Clinton Administration as Assistant Director for International Affairs in the Office of Science and Technology Policy. In this position, Dr. Schweitzer was responsible for providing scientific and technological policy advice and analysis for Al Gore, President Clinton, and President Clinton's Science Advisor, and for coordinating the U.S. government's international science and technology cooperative initiatives.

Dr. Schweitzer's work has been fueled by his desire to introduce a stronger set of ethics into American efforts to improve the human condition worldwide. He has been instrumental in designing programs that demonstrate how third world development and protecting our resources are compatible goals. His vision is to inspire a framework that ensures that humans can grow and prosper indefinitely in a healthy environment.

Dr. Schweitzer earned his Ph.D. from Scripps Institution of Oceanography at the University of California, San Diego.

To learn more about Dr Schweitzer, you can visit his website at http://www.jeffschweitzer.com.

INDEX

A

activities, calorie-burning capacity, 33. *See also* exercise

adipose tissue. *See* body fat

aerobic respiration, 5

"afterburn" effect, of interval training, 34

age

  basal metabolic rate and, 13

  weight and, 52

anabolism, 5

anti-inflammatory foods, diet myths regarding, 51–52

appetite. *See* satiety response

arthritis, 45, 46

Atkins Diet, 31

ATP, 5

B

balanced diet, 4, 30

basal metabolic rate, 12–13

bedtime, eating prior to, 2–4

behaviors and habits

  regarding exercise, 34, 35–36

  regarding food. *see* eating habits

  reinforcement of, 22

  reprogramming, 19–20

  self-analysis of, 14

belly fat diet myth, 50–51

Betty (case history), 37–38

birth defects, 46

blood sugar levels, 44, 51

blood volume, 12

body composition, 6, 7–8, 11–12, 13, 52

J
Jenny Craig diet plan, 31
joints, excess weight and, 45
juice, vs. fruit, 25, 26

K
kilocalories. *See* calories

L
LDL (low density lipoprotein), 48
legumes, 25
leptin, 44
Livestrong Calorie Tracker, 60
low fat vs. low calorie diet myth, 47
low-energy-density foods, 24–25, 30

M
Mary (case history), 16–17
meal planning, 23
Meal Snap, 60
meal timing, 2–4. *See also* portion sizes
medications, satiety response and, 8
meditation, 40
Mediterranean diet/panty, 27–29, 57
men
    basal metabolic rate, 13
    daily calorie intake guidelines, 9
mental imagery, 16–17. *See also* psychological factors
metabolism, 4–5, 12–13, 52
mindful eating, 24
mobile app resources, 60
mono-unsaturated fats, 48
motivation, 37. *See also* commitment
muscle tissue, 7, 11–12
My Fitness Pal, 59
My Recipes, 57
My Yoga Online, 58
myths, about weight loss, 43–53

respiration, 5
restaurant meals, 23
Restructure Your Relationship with Food weight loss rule, 39–41, 55
RunKeeper, 60

S
satiety response
   eating habits and, 21
   fad diets and, 30–32
   fiber and, 25
   genetics and, 7
   myths regarding, 44
   water consumption and, 23–24
saturated fats, 48, 49
Schweitzer, Jeff, 65
seeds, 29
self-analysis, 14–16, 37. *See also* fitness tools
self-hypnosis, 19, 40
serial dieting, x
sexual activity, 47, 53
sleep apnea, 46
sleep interruptions, 3
smoking, 8, 45
snacks, suggestions for, 27
social conventions, around food, 21
South Beach diet plan, 31–32
spices, 29
sports, calorie-burning capacity, 33
stress
   cortisol link, 51
   management of, 16–17, 40
stroke, 45
Super Slow exercise programs, 35–36, 58
supplements, ix, 43–44

T
temperature, 53

www.ingramcontent.com/pod-product-compliance
Lightning Source LLC
Chambersburg PA
CBHW022125280326
41933CB00007B/548